HIGH PERFORMANCE, FRAGILE BALANCE

A MEMOIR OF AMBITION, MENTAL HEALTH AND RECOVERY

KRISHNAPAL SINGH

Made with ♥ on the Notion Press Platform
www.notionpress.com

Dedicated to my family, friends, colleagues, and everyone who has played a part in shaping me as a person throughout this journey.

Contents

Preface

I never imagined I would write a book about mental illness. In 2022, my life took an unexpected turn. At the time, neither I nor my family fully understood what was happening. We were confused, worried, and searching for answers. Like many people facing a mental health crisis for the first time, we tried to make sense of an experience that seemed impossible to explain. Over the next few years, our lives were shaped by uncertainty, recovery, setbacks, and profound learning. In 2025, I was formally diagnosed with bipolar disorder. The diagnosis provided clarity, but it also marked the beginning of a new chapter—one dedicated to understanding myself and the journey my family and I had already traveled. This book is my attempt to tell that story honestly. It is not a medical guide or a collection of expert advice. It is a deeply personal account of what happened, how it affected the people I love, and what I learned along the way.I chose to write this book because mental illness is still frequently misunderstood and rarely discussed openly. If my experiences help even one person feel less alone, or help a family better understand what a loved one is enduring, then sharing this story will have been worthwhile.

— Krishna Pal Singh

Acknowledgements

This book is the result of a journey that I could not have completed alone. My heartfelt thanks to my family for their love, patience, unwavering support through both the good times and difficult ones.

To my friends, colleagues, mentors, and the mental health professionals who guided me along the way, thank you for your encouragement, understanding, and belief in me when i needed it most.

Finally, thank you to everyone who has been part of my journey and helped shape me into the person I am today.

With gratitude,
Krishnapal Singh

1
The First Crack

For most of my life, I believed that discipline could solve almost anything. Engineering problems responded to effort. Career growth followed persistence. Stability felt like something that could be earned and systematically maintained. It took me years to realize that mental illness does not follow the same rules.

Work had structure. Engineering problems had boundaries. Inputs and outputs were visible. If I worked consistently, outcomes generally followed. Over time, that way of thinking became not just professional, but personal.

Then came COVID-19.

Work moved into the home. Days became continuous, bleeding into one another. Meetings stretched late into the night. The boundary between work and rest began to blur, then vanished entirely. Sleep started to change during this period.

At first, it was subtle—going to bed later, waking up slightly less rested. I did not see it as a problem. It felt like part of the baseline adjustment everyone was going through. There was always a logical reason to stay up a little longer: work items, global messages, unfinished tasks.

Around this time, I received an internal transfer opportunity to the United States, near Boston. It was a major career milestone. While I focused intently on the professional opportunity and the logistics of the move, my wife, Raksha, carried much of the emotional and logistical burden. She was the one thinking about how we would rebuild our daily lives in an entirely new country with a young child—our son was still under two years old.

Looking back, the relocation was as much her journey as it was mine, if not more. The move felt like progress. It was structured and forward-looking. But beneath the surface, my sleep remained unstable.

August 2022

In August, something changed in a way I could not easily explain. My sleep had become increasingly irregular, and my thinking began to feel less anchored than usual.

I started noticing interpretations that were uncommon for me. For example, when bank-related text messages arrived on my phone, I would briefly question whether they were part of some internal administrative process beyond what I could see directly—whether different parts of a hidden system were communicating in a way that I was not fully aware of. There were also moments when I felt an uneasy sensation that I was being observed or recorded.

These thoughts were not constant, nor were they fully formed. They would appear, hover, and pass, flashing most vividly during periods of severe sleep deprivation and mental fatigue.I did not share these experiences widely at the time. I tried to rationalize them as standard stress, overwork, or a temporary lack of rest. Outwardly, I continued functioning normally in daily life and at work.

October 2022 — Sehore

In October, we travelled to Sehore for a family function. This is where the first major physical collapse occurred. I found myself entirely unable to sleep through the night.

My body felt restless, vibrating and overstimulated. The next day, the physical toll manifested as elevated blood pressure, severe palpitations, and intense agitation. Emotionally, I was unstable and highly reactive.

The unusual thoughts from August were no longer the main feature; instead, the raw lack of sleep and physical stress intensified everything else. It felt as though my internal system had broken past its operational limits.

We sought immediate medical help. I was prescribed Lorazepam, which finally allowed me to sleep. With rest, the intensity of the symptoms reduced quickly. Within a short time, the situation appeared to stabilize.

Afterward, life resumed its forward trajectory. The plan to move to the United States continued exactly as before. The opportunity remained fully intact. Nothing yet suggested a long-term disruption. I did not understand then that August and October were not isolated incidents. They were part of the same unfolding pattern. I simply did not have the language for it yet.

2

Arrival, Normalcy, and the First Collapse

We moved to the United States in late 2022.

Our new home near Boston felt structured and orderly in a way that was immediately noticeable. After months of travel, adjustment, and quiet uncertainty, that order felt grounding. It represented the stability we wanted professionally, personally, and for our family.We began our transition in temporary housing during the peak of winter.

The biting cold shaped everything in those early days. Simple routines required immense effort. Stepping outside, running errands, and executing small daily movements felt significantly heavier than before.Our son was still under two years old.

Most of our attention naturally centered around his adjustment—his sleep, his comfort, and his ability to settle into a completely unfamiliar environment. As parents, we were in a constant state of practical problem-solving.

Work began in parallel. There was onboarding, absorbing new team dynamics, and navigating fresh expectations. I focused heavily on establishing continuity. After a major international relocation, it felt vital to demonstrate stability and performance without a single interruption.

From the outside, everything was functioning seamlessly. Internally, my sleep was still fracturing. It had never truly returned to what it was before the disruptions began. Some nights were fragmented; some mornings felt entirely un-restorative. I attributed this to jet lag, environmental changes, and the natural strain of relocation. There was no single moment that felt like a red flag—only a quiet continuity of the earlier disruptions.

Gradually, we settled into a predictable routine. We moved out of temporary housing. Work stabilized. Daily life became reliable. The urgency of the relocation began to fade. From a distance, this phase would have looked like a complete recovery. In many ways, it was.

But the stability was incomplete. My sleep remained lighter than it used to be. My energy levels swung, and my emotional responses were slightly less even, though still within a range that could be explained away individually. Nothing felt connected.

Then, we took a family trip to Florida. It was meant to be a true break—warm weather, dedicated family time, and distance from routine pressures. We went to Orlando, exploring places like Walt Disney World. For a few days, life felt lighter.

During this trip, I made the decision to stop my medication. It did not feel significant at the time. It felt temporary and almost procedural—a short interruption during travel that surely wouldn't affect my baseline stability. Almost immediately, my sleep began to shift.It wasn't dramatic. It didn't loudly demand attention. It was subtle—slightly lighter rest, slightly less physical recovery, a creeping sense that my sleep was no longer whole. I noticed it, but I didn't interpret it for what it was.

We returned to our home in Acton, near Boston, and resumed normal life. But my sleep did not return to baseline. A quiet instability remained in the house.Then, things escalated with terrifying speed.My internal state and behavior began to change in ways that became visible to those around me. What I was experiencing internally and what others observed from the outside began to sharply diverge. Eventually, I reached a terrifying point of clarity where I recognized that something was no longer under my control.

I called emergency services myself. The dispatchers asked me heavy, grounding questions:

Did I have intentions to hurt someone else?

Did I feel like hurting myself?

I was taken by ambulance to a nearby medical hospital.

While I experienced the crisis from the deep interior of the illness, my wife experienced it entirely from the outside—frantically trying to understand what was happening to her husband while caring for our young son in a foreign country, far away from our family support systems. Some of my memories from that period are fragmented, but I know with certainty that she carried far more of the burden than I could fully appreciate at the time.

What followed was no longer something that could be explained away as stress, adjustment, or simple fatigue. My functioning collapsed. My speech became minimal. My physical movement and responsiveness became severely impaired. It felt as though my access to basic human expression had been abruptly switched off.

At the hospital, multiple clinicians evaluated me. Numerous investigations were conducted. The focus shifted quickly to a severe functional state that required urgent psychiatric intervention.A psychiatrist diagnosed me with catatonia. My medications were adjusted, and I was started on Quetiapine.

Over time, there was a gradual, halting recovery—first my sleep returned, then my responsiveness, and finally, my communication.

During this period, there were ongoing discussions with clinicians trying to understand the overarching pattern across the months: the sleep disruptions, the emotional variability, the behavioral shifts, and the repeated episodes that refused to fit neatly into isolated explanations.

At that stage, there was still no single, unified understanding. I was recovering, but I was not yet understanding.Florida had felt like a break. In reality, it had been the catalyst for a collapse that had been forming quietly for months.

3

Recovery Without Clarity

After leaving the medical hospital, the immediate goal was simple: stabilize and recover. Sleep returned first, followed by energy, and then the ability to function in small, ordinary ways again— speaking, walking, and engaging in daily routines.

On the surface, the acute crisis had passed. My medications were adjusted during this period, including the Quetiapine, with a strict focus on preventing another acute episode and maintaining our hard-won stability.

There was also ongoing follow-up with the psychiatrist who had diagnosed the catatonia. I met with him once a month, paying around $50 per session. Our discussions were not only medical but interpretive—we were trying to map out the trajectory of what had happened.

At one point, he told me that my condition might be long-term, and that I may need to continue medications like Lorazepam for a prolonged period, possibly indefinitely. He also suggested a coping mechanism: if certain situations or people triggered acute stress, I should try not to engage emotionally in the moment. He described it as placing the emotional response into a "box" during the interaction, to be reopened and revisited later when I was alone. He suggested that if I could do this consistently, future interactions might feel easier over time.

Alongside medical care, deep personal decisions were being discussed at home, including whether moving back to India would be better for my long-term stability.

In parallel, life slowly resumed. We traveled back to India in December 2023. On December 12th, I went to Gwalior. On December 15th, we traveled to Sehore for a family function. During this hectic period of travel and family gatherings, we unfortunately missed maintaining our medication continuity. That small disruption proved to be critical.

My sleep quickly became unstable again. Within a short time, my mental state began to shift. What started as a mild imbalance gradually escalated into a much more noticeable episode. The situation worsened significantly when I returned to Gwalior.

My behavior became aggressive toward family members, and my emotional regulation shattered. Despite the intensity of the situation, my family continued to support me unconditionally, relying on their spiritual coping mechanisms and providing constant care throughout the episode. Eventually, things were stabilized again through targeted medical intervention and a strict return to routine.

On January 20th, we moved back to the United States, returning to our home in Acton. For about a month, things appeared stable again. But underneath, the pattern was quietly re-emerging.

4

The Return of Instability

I remained stable for nearly a month after our return. Work had resumed, life had routines again, and there was a comforting sense that things had finally settled after the long, grueling cycle of disruption, hospitalization, and recovery. But in the third week of February, something shifted.

I happened to see the name of a friend in a work-related thread. It triggered an emotional response that was warm, positive, and deeply personal. In that immediate moment, I became highly emotionally activated. I began sending messages in corporate work channels that were completely irrelevant to the professional context.

From the inside, it didn't feel disruptive at all. It felt like genuine connection, profound involvement, and an urgent need to engage with others. But the sheer volume and content of the messages were entirely misaligned with professional boundaries.

This quickly became visible to leadership. Human Resources and my managers intervened. My manager spoke to me directly, explaining clearly that my actions were affecting my professional credibility. At the time, I agreed with him completely and reassured him that it would not happen again. But the pattern repeated.

Despite my best intentions and conscious awareness, I was unable to control the overwhelming urge to respond and engage in the exact same manner. More out-of-context messages followed. Human Resources stepped in once more. This time, the communication was formal. I received an email to my personal account stating that their primary concern was my health and well-being, and outlining the support resources available to me.

Eventually, due to my repeated inability to comply with communication boundaries—specifically around messaging certain employees—I was informed that my systems would be deactivated and I would be placed on paid administrative leave. I accepted it at the time as a necessary step. Soon after, I chose to seek medical help.

I checked back into the same nearby medical hospital. This time, my state settled quickly. Within a single day, the acute emotional intensity reduced significantly. My medication regimen was reviewed, and Lorazepam was systematically discontinued. Over the next two to three clinical sessions, the psychiatrist evaluated my condition and determined that I was stable enough from a psychiatric standpoint to be transitioned.

One of the vital observations made by the medical team was that I had not been fully communicating the extent of my work-related and emotional experiences with my wife. They emphasized that total transparency at home would be essential for my ongoing stability.

I was moved to a structured inpatient setting within the psychiatric unit, an environment I found surprisingly organized and deeply supportive. There was a rigid daily schedule: therapy sessions, group activities, art room sessions, daytime yoga, evening walks, and structured discussions centered on coping skills like Cognitive Behavioral Therapy (CBT) and substance management. The environment felt profoundly stabilizing.

The psychiatrist recommended an extended stay of about one more week. After nearly two weeks in total, I was discharged with official documentation stating that I was fit to return to work. My diagnosis at that time was documented as Major Depressive Disorder (MDD). I returned to work after that period.

For about a month, things functioned smoothly again. But by July, I started feeling the heavy, familiar return of depressive symptoms. One afternoon, my wife and I were sitting in our community area. She was commenting on how peaceful and beautiful the surroundings felt. At that exact moment, I was internally consumed by thoughts of stepping away from my career entirely and taking an extended medical break.

I spoke to a close friend about it, and he supported the idea. I then approached my manager and shared that I was considering a medical leave of six months or more, after which I would reassess whether I should return to work in Hyderabad or near Boston.After internal discussions, coordination with leadership, and formal approvals—including communication that went up to the VP level—the leave was approved.

I officially stepped away from work on August 10. Before leaving, I closed down our rented home, packed our lives, and sold my car, marking a definitive end to that chapter. I returned to India to begin a longer, intentional period of recovery and reset.

5

The Long Pause

I returned to India on medical leave.

This time, the focus was not on recovering from a single, isolated episode, but on trying to regain basic stability over a prolonged stretch of time. The pressure of work was entirely gone. External expectations had vanished. Life became slower, narrower, and deeply contained.

My medical leave continued until February 13, 2025. During this period, I consulted a doctor who prescribed specialized medication for my sleep and anxiety. My sleep requirements increased significantly—I was often sleeping around 12 hours a day. The days became long, quiet stretches of rest, with very little activity in between. On most days, I did not do much beyond staying at home or visiting relatives.

Emotionally, this was one of the lowest phases of my entire life.

I battled persistent depression, a total lack of motivation, and a crushing sense of being unable to engage with the world in a meaningful way. It felt less like active recovery and more like being permanently paused in place.

During this heavy period, my wife consistently became the source of momentum for our family. When I struggled to see any progress, she continued to move life forward, creating a protective layer of stability around me until I was capable of participating in it again.

There were a few external events that stood out during this time. One was my sister-in-law's wedding in early February. Despite my state, I was able to participate, and I genuinely enjoyed those days. For a short window, there was lightness, true connection, and presence. But that feeling did not outlast the event.

On February 14, 2025, I officially returned to work at our office in Hyderabad.

My manager and colleagues welcomed me back with incredible warmth. For a while, things felt stable again. Work provided routine, and routine provided direction. This stability sustained itself for several months. But in early July, the pattern began to shift once more.

My sleep became severely disturbed, and I found myself spending excessive hours reading and intensely engaging with work-related content across various AI tools and professional discussions. It did not feel harmful at first—it felt like pure curiosity and high engagement—but it was gradually fracturing my internal balance.

My wife noticed the early signs of change and became deeply concerned. She proactively informed my manager that my health did not seem stable. My manager was incredibly supportive and suggested an immediate evaluation at a nearby hospital in Hyderabad. I went there accompanied by my wife and close friends from work.

During that consultation, I described everything that had happened since 2022 in meticulous detail. It was the very first time the entire timeline had been spoken aloud, sequentially, in a single room.

After evaluating the full history, the psychiatrist diagnosed me with Bipolar Disorder.

My treatment plan was changed significantly. I was immediately started on Lithium at 450 mg. What followed was a gradual, grounding return to stability. Over the next few weeks, my mood began to settle.

Within about three weeks, I felt a noticeable, profound shift back toward my true baseline. More than the medication itself, what stood out during this period was the safety net of support around me—my wife, friends, and colleagues who stayed deeply involved and present through the entire transition. By the end of this phase, life had become structured again. But this time, I had a much clearer understanding: stability was not accidental. It had to be maintained deliberately, especially now that the patterns had finally revealed themselves.

6

Joy, Stability, and the Return of the Cycle

We were expecting our second child when I was formally diagnosed with bipolar disorder.

Even with the weight of that new diagnosis, life continued forward in parallel. There was treatment, constant adjustment, and a collective effort to rebuild stability while simultaneously preparing to welcome a new life into our home.

On December 21, 2025, our daughter, Aarna, was born.

The months that followed should have been defined solely by the pure joy of welcoming a daughter. Instead, my wife was forced to balance the exhausting demands of a newborn, an energetic young son, and the constant, looming uncertainty of my health.

Looking back, I have a much deeper appreciation for the immense strength that required of her. Aarna's arrival brought deep joy. In the middle of years characterized by disruption, hospital visits, medication adjustments, and anxiety, her presence felt profoundly grounding. For a while, life felt whole again in a way it hadn't for a very long time.

Shortly after, we shifted back into celebratory family milestones. On February 1, 2026, we celebrated our elder son Advait's fifth birthday in Hyderabad. The entire family came together. It was a happy, deeply connected celebration, and those days felt profoundly stable and meaningful.

During this period, I was also in regular discussions with my doctor regarding long-term treatment protocols. One of our conversations centered around whether my Lithium dosage could eventually be reduced or discontinued entirely if I managed to remain fully stable for about a year.

For a while, things did remain entirely stable. Work felt manageable, family life felt beautifully structured, and there was a creeping sense that the difficult cycles were finally behind us—or at least firmly under control. But by the end of March 2026, the familiar pattern began to whisper again.

I found myself spending increased amounts of time reading work-related material on AI tools, specifically fixating on appraisal cycles and corporate discussions. Gradually, my sleep began to fracture.

My wife noticed the early warning signs immediately, just as she had in earlier episodes. We promptly consulted our doctor. Initially, the clinical assessment was that it looked like an isolated sleep disturbance rather than a full manic relapse. However, as the symptoms persisted over the following days, we sought further evaluation from another doctor within the same hospital system.My medication was adjusted immediately. My Lithium dosage was increased significantly, adding Lithosun 800 mg at night alongside Lithocent 450 mg in the morning.

By this point, however, the momentum of the episode had already escalated past the point of early intervention. I began sending emails at work despite being on baby bonding leave. Some of these communications were intense, high-velocity, and entirely out of context, including messages fired off over weekends to team members and a close colleague. Despite my friends at work and my manager attempting to step in and gently intervene, I was simply not capable of stopping the behavior during that period. It became undeniably clear that this was another manic episode.

We went to the hospital again. I was given an injection as part of our acute stabilization protocol. Over the following weeks, my condition gradually improved, and within about three weeks, I returned once more to a stable baseline.

Following my recovery, my work assignment was thoughtfully adjusted to a more research-oriented project, explicitly taking into account the medical need for a lower-stress, highly structured environment.

Since then, I have been in a much more stable phase—strongly supported by regular treatment, my family, and ongoing medical oversight.

At this point in my journey, the pattern is no longer abstract or confusing. It is visible, repeated, and thoroughly understood. I am learning, slowly and deliberately, what it means to live with it, rather than simply reacting to it after the damage is done.

7

Living With the Balance

One of the greatest lessons this journey has taught me is that stability does not happen by accident.

For a long time, I viewed each psychiatric episode as a completely separate, unfortunate event. It was only over time that I began to see the systemic connections. The most consistent, undeniable pattern was the direct, mathematical relationship between my sleep and my mental health.

Today, protecting my sleep is the single most important component of my treatment plan. I maintain a strict sleep schedule, going to bed around 10:00 PM and waking up between 6:00 and 7:00 AM. I have learned the hard way that even minor disruptions in sleep have compounding consequences that are not immediately visible.

Alongside sleep, daily routine has become my scaffolding. My therapist and doctors have encouraged me to anchor myself in regular habits: waking up at the exact same time, eating meals at fixed intervals, and engaging in moderate physical exercise like swimming. These activities may seem simple from the outside, but together they provide the structural boundaries that support internal stability.

I have also learned the profound value of slowing down and intentionally creating space for recovery. My therapist suggested reading physical books as a practical way to reduce cognitive stress and shift my attention away from constant digital stimulation. Journaling has been another vital practice recommended by my medical team; writing down my daily thoughts and physical metrics helps me recognize shifts in energy that might otherwise go unnoticed.

Since May 2026, I have been attending therapy sessions regularly in Hyderabad. Therapy has given me the behavioral tools to better understand my emotions, manage acute stress, and identify specific situations that threaten my mental well-being. It has also forced me to think much more deliberately about true work-life balance.

Work remains incredibly important to me, but I no longer view professional success as something that should ever come at the expense of my health. Maintaining rigid boundaries, protecting personal time, and creating uncompromised space for rest are now core components of how I define long-term career sustainability.

Another invaluable lesson is that managing bipolar disorder is not a solo endeavor. My wife has been the anchor of this entire journey.

Over the years, she learned to recognize the subtle changes in my behavior and sleep patterns that I was entirely blind to. She stood beside me through ambulance rides, psychiatric wards, deep depressions, manic instabilities, and the long, grueling stretches of recovery. Many of the crucial decisions that protected my life happened simply because she noticed something was wrong and acted before the situation could worsen. This story is written from my perspective, but I know it would have a very different, much darker ending without her support, patience, and resilience.

If there is one message I want readers to take away from these pages, it is this: medication matters.

For a long time, I secretly hoped that clinical insight and intellectual understanding of the condition would be enough to keep me safe. My experiences shattered that illusion. Insight is important, therapy is vital, and family support is indispensable—but consistent medication is the chemical foundation of stability. Accepting psychiatric treatment was not a sign of weakness or a failure of discipline. It was the single most courageous step toward living a full, stable life.

I do not know exactly what the future holds. Bipolar disorder is a chronic condition that requires lifetime attention and meticulous care. But I am no longer fighting it from a place of confusion.

I understand the patterns clearly now. I know the value of sleep, routine, treatment, and community. Most importantly, I understand that stability is not a permanent state you achieve—it is something you actively protect, day after day. The balance may be fragile, but it is infinitely worth protecting.

Epilogue: Looking Forward

When I look back at the years chronicled in this book, what stands out most vividly is not the hospitalizations, the clinical diagnoses, or the episodes. It is the beautiful, ordinary life that stubbornly continued around them.

There were birthdays celebrated with cake, warm family gatherings, complex engineering projects delivered, school milestones, and quiet everyday routines.

My life was never entirely defined by illness, and it was never entirely free from it either. Today, I continue to work as an engineer at the same company where I began my career nearly fifteen years ago. For much of that time, I measured my worth exclusively through professional achievement and corporate leveling. While work remains deeply fulfilling, I am still working on measuring the true meaning of success.

Today, success means being healthy. It means being fully present for my family. It means being able to contribute meaningfully at work without breaking myself.

One of the greatest transformations on this journey has occurred within my marriage. What began as love has gradually evolved into something far deeper and more resilient: true compassion. Through every episode, hospitalization, and recovery, my wife carried invisible responsibilities. Many of the interventions that preserved my health occurred simply because she recognized the warning signs before I did.

Being a father has also completely reshaped my perspective. Advait and Aarna are still so young, and I want more than anything to be a steady, present force in their lives. I want them to grow up knowing that asking for help is a profound act of strength, and that mental health deserves the exact same attention, care, and respect as physical health.

Receiving a formal diagnosis of bipolar disorder did not instantly solve all my problems, but it gave me an invaluable gift: understanding. Today, I recognize my shifting moods better, respect the absolute necessity of sleep, and pay close, analytical attention to changes in my thinking, energy, and behavior. I still experience worry about future episodes, particularly how they might impact my family and my career. But I have learned to channel that anxiety into focusing strictly on what I can actively control: my medication compliance, my sleep hygiene, my daily routine, my therapy sessions, my physical exercise, and early medical intervention the moment something feels off-balance.

I ultimately decided to write this book because mental illness remains deeply misunderstood by so many. I grew up in Gwalior, and while public awareness is steadily improving, access to quality mental health care and open, shame-free conversations about psychiatric conditions still desperately need to improve within our communities. If these chapters help even one person seek clinical help a little earlier, better understand a struggling loved one, or feel a little less isolated in their own darkness, then sharing my story openly will have been worth every word.

Bipolar disorder is an undeniable part of my life, but it is not the whole story. I am an engineer. I am a husband. I am a father. And I am a human being, still learning every single day.

The future will inevitably bring both beautiful stability and unexpected challenges. What gives me confidence today is not the illusion that difficult times will never return. It is the grounding knowledge that I understand my condition, I am surrounded by an unwavering safety net of support, and I know exactly what I must do to protect the balance.

For now, that is enough.

www.ingramcontent.com/pod-product-compliance
Lightning Source LLC
LaVergne TN
LVHW090337210926
848480LV00004B/1444
* 9 7 9 8 9 0 5 1 0 7 7 2 6 *